the healthy

You owe it to yourself to take this handbook to heart. For coronary heart disease is a woman's concern. Every woman's concern. It is not something that only affects your husband, your father, your brother, your son. This handbook tells you why you should be concerned about your own heart health, and what you can do to prevent coronary disease. A little prevention can have a big payoff — a longer, healthier, more active life.

Each year, 245,000 women die of coronary heart disease, making it the number one killer of American women. Another 90,000 women die each year of stroke. Although death rates from coronary heart disease and stroke have declined in recent years, these conditions still rank first and third, respectively, as causes of death for women.

Overall, about 10 million American women of all ages suffer from heart disease. One in ten women 45 to 64 years of age has some form of heart disease, and this increases to one in four women over 65. Each year, one-half million women suffer heart attacks. Cardiovascular diseases and their prevention, therefore, are pressing personal concerns for every woman.

heart

what are cardiovascular diseases?

Cardiovascular diseases are diseases of the heart and blood vessel system, such as coronary heart disease, heart attack, high blood pressure, stroke, angina (chest pain), and rheumatic heart disease. Coronary heart disease — the primary subject of this handbook — is a disease of the blood vessels of the heart that causes heart attacks. A heart attack happens when an artery becomes blocked, preventing oxygen and nutrients from getting to the heart. A stroke results from a lack of blood to the brain, or in some cases, bleeding in the brain.

who gets cardiovascular diseases?

Some women have more "risk factors" for cardiovascular diseases than others. Risk factors are
traits or habits that make a person more likely to
develop a disease. Some risk factors for heart-
related problems cannot be changed, but others
can be. The three major risk factors for cardiovascular disease that you can do something about are
cigarette smoking, high blood pressure, and high
blood cholesterol. Other risk factors, such as
overweight, diabetes, and physical inactivity, also
are conditions you have some control over. Although growing older is a risk factor that cannot
be changed, it is important to realize that other
risks can be reduced at any age. This handbook
identifies some key risk factors that you can control,
and suggests changes in living habits to lessen your
chances of developing cardiovascular diseases.

Some groups of women are more likely to develop
cardiovascular diseases than other groups. Black
women are 24 percent more likely to die of coronary heart disease than white women, and their
death rate for stroke is 83 percent higher. Older
women have a greater chance of developing cardiovascular diseases than younger women, partly
because the tendency to have heart-related problems increases with age. Older women, for
example, are more likely to develop high blood
pressure and high blood cholesterol levels, to be
diabetic, to be overweight, and to exercise less than
younger women. Also, after menopause, women

are more apt to get cardiovascular diseases, in part because their bodies produce less estrogen. Women who have had early menopause, either naturally or by means of a hysterectomy, are twice as likely to develop coronary heart disease as women of the same age who have not begun menopause.

While any one risk factor will raise your chances of developing heart-related problems, the more risk factors you have, the more concerned you should be about prevention. If you smoke cigarettes and have high blood pressure, for example, your chance of developing coronary heart disease goes up dramatically. Having all three major changeable risk factors — smoking, high blood pressure, and high blood cholesterol — can boost your risk to eight times that of women who have no risk factors.

Changing habits isn't easy — but experience shows that it works. As Americans have learned to control blood pressure and make healthful changes in their eating, smoking, and exercise habits, death rates for heart attack and stroke have dropped dramatically. Between 1970 and 1988, the death rate for women from coronary heart disease was cut in half. During the same period, the death rate for stroke went down 55 percent.

Cardiovascular diseases remain the leading cause of death for American women. But the message is clear: by taking an active role in your own heart health, you can make a difference. Beginning with the chapter on "Self-Help Strategies for a Healthy Heart," this handbook supplies a number of practical tips to help you get started. Also, for information about other organizations and materials available to help you, see "Resources for a Healthy Heart" on page 81.

major
risk factors

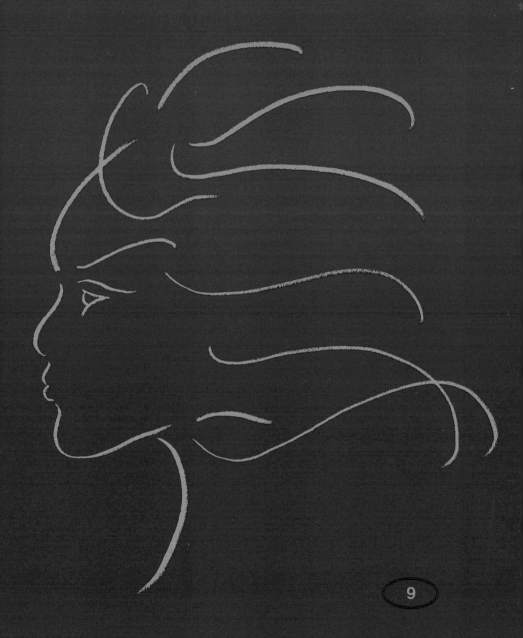

major risk factors

SMOKING

Cigarette smoking has been described as "the most important individual health risk in this country." Approximately 26 million American women smoke. Although the smoking rate for women dropped 8 percent between 1965 and 1988, women who smoke today are apt to smoke more heavily than they did in the past.

Surprising as it may seem, smoking by women in the United States causes almost as many deaths from heart disease as from lung cancer. Women who smoke are two to six times as likely to suffer a heart attack as nonsmoking women, and the risk increases with the number of cigarettes smoked per day. Smoking also boosts the risk of stroke.

Cardiovascular diseases are not the only health risks for women who smoke. Cigarette smoking greatly increases the chances that a woman will develop lung cancer. In fact, the lung cancer death rate for women is now higher than the death rate for breast cancer, the chief cause of cancer deaths in women for many years. Cigarette smoking is also linked with cancers of the mouth, larynx, esophagus, urinary tract, kidney, pancreas, and cervix. Smoking also causes 80 percent of cases of chronic obstructive lung disease, which includes bronchitis and emphysema.

small dose, big benefit

If you are one of the 3 million older Americans with a type of high blood pressure called isolated systolic hypertension (ISH), there is good news. A recent study shows that treating ISH with a low dose of a common blood pressure-lowering drug, a diuretic called cholorthalidone, cut the risk of stroke by more than one-third, and reduced the risk of coronary heart disease by 27 percent. The dose of the diuretic used in the study was only half of the smallest dose usually first given to patients. One in five patients also took a low dose of a second drug, a beta-blocker, to help lower their blood pressure.

If you have ISH and are already doing well on another type of blood pressure-lowering drug, you should not necessarily switch medicines. But you may want to discuss with your doctor whether the treatment used successfully in this study might work for you.

Smoking is also linked to a number of reproductive problems. Women who smoke are more apt to have problems getting pregnant and to begin menopause at a slightly younger age. Further, cigarette use during pregnancy poses serious risks for the unborn. Babies of women who smoked during pregnancy tend to weigh less at birth than babies of nonsmokers. Smoking while pregnant also increases risks of bleeding, miscarriage, premature delivery, stillbirth, and sudden infant death syndrome, or "crib death." Moreover, young children who are exposed to a parent's cigarette smoke have more lung and ear infections.

There is simply no "safe way" to smoke. Although low-tar and -nicotine cigarettes may reduce the lung cancer risk to some extent, they do not lessen the risks of heart diseases or other smoking-related diseases. The only safe and healthful course is not to smoke at all.

HIGH BLOOD PRESSURE

High blood pressure, also known as hypertension, is another major risk factor for coronary heart diseases and the most important risk factor for stroke. Even slightly high levels double the risk. High blood pressure also boosts the chances of developing kidney disease.

Nearly 58 million Americans have high blood pressure, and about half of them are women. Older women have a higher risk, with more than half of all women over the age of 55 suffering from this condition. High blood pressure is more common and more severe in black women than it is in white women. Use of birth control pills can contribute to high blood pressure in some women.

Blood pressure is the amount of force exerted by the blood against the walls of the arteries. Everyone has to have some blood pressure, so that blood can get to the body's organs and muscles. Usually, blood pressure is expressed as two numbers, such as 120/80, and is measured in millimeters of mercury (mmHg). The first number is the systolic blood pressure, the force used when the heart beats. The second number, or diastolic blood pressure, is the pressure that exists in the arteries between heartbeats. Depending on your activities, blood pressure may move up or down in the course of a day. Blood pressure is considered high when it stays above normal levels over a period of time.

High blood pressure is sometimes called the "silent killer" because most people have it without feeling sick. Therefore, it is important to have it checked each time you see your doctor or other health professional. Blood pressure can be easily measured by means of the familiar stethoscope and inflatable cuff placed around one arm. However, since blood pressure changes so often and is affected by many factors, your health professional should check it on several different days before deciding if your blood pressure is too high. If your blood pressure stays at 140/90 mmHg or above, you have high blood pressure.

Although high blood pressure can rarely be cured, it can be controlled with proper treatment. If your blood pressure is not too high, you may be able to control it entirely through weight loss if you are overweight, regular exercise, and cutting down on alcohol, table salt, and sodium. (Sodium is an ingredient in salt that is found in many packaged foods, baking soda, and some antacids.)

However, if your blood pressure remains high, your doctor will probably prescribe medicine in addition to the above changes. The amount you take may be gradually reduced, especially if you are successful with the changes you make in your lifestyle. While few people like the idea of taking any medicine for a long time, the treatment benefits are real and will reduce the risk of stroke, heart attack, and kidney disease. If you are pre-scribed a drug to control high blood pressure and find you have any uncomfortable side effects, ask your doctor about changing the dosage or possibly switching to another type of medicine.

During pregnancy, some women develop high blood pressure for the first time. Between 10 and 20 percent of first-time mothers develop a high blood pressure problem during pregnancy called preeclampsia. Other women who already have high blood pressure may find that it worsens during pregnancy. If untreated, these conditions can be life-threatening to both mother and baby. Since a woman can feel perfectly normal and still have one of these conditions, it is important to get regular prenatal checkups so that your doctor can discover and treat a possible high blood pressure problem.

HIGH BLOOD CHOLESTEROL

High blood cholesterol is a third important risk factor for coronary heart diseases that you can do something about. Although young women tend to have lower cholesterol levels than young men, between the ages of 45 and 55, women's cholesterol levels begin to rise higher than men's.

After age 55, the gap between women and men becomes still wider. Today, about one-third of American women have blood cholesterol levels high enough to pose a serious risk for coronary heart diseases. The higher your blood cholesterol level, the higher your heart disease risk. For all adults, a desirable blood cholesterol level is less than 200 mg/dL. A level of 240 mg/dL or above is considered "high" blood cholesterol. But even levels in the "borderline-high" category (200-239 mg/dL) boost the risk of heart disease.

cholesterol: the age factor

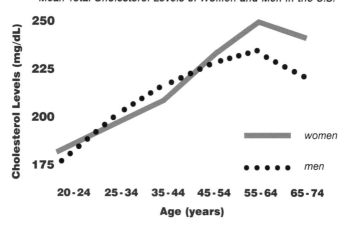

Mean Total Cholesterol Levels of Women and Men in the U.S.

Cholesterol Levels (mg/dL)

250 — 225 — 200 — 175

20-24 25-34 35-44 45-54 55-64 65-74

Age (years)

—— women

• • • • • men

Source: National Health and Nutrition Examination Survey (1976-80)

The body needs cholesterol to function normally. It is found in all foods that come from animals — that is, all meats and dairy products. However, the body can make all of the cholesterol that it needs. Over a period of years, extra cholesterol and fat circulating in the blood settle on the inner walls of the arteries that supply blood to the heart. These deposits make the arteries narrower and narrower. As a result, less blood gets to the heart and the risk of coronary heart disease increases.

Ask your health professional to check your blood cholesterol level once every 5 years. This simple test involves taking a small blood sample and measuring the amount of cholesterol. The cholesterol level is expressed as, for example, "215 mg/dL" or 215 milligrams of cholesterol per deciliter of blood. Be sure to ask what your cholesterol number is and whether you should take steps to lower it. Before age 45, the total blood cholesterol level of women averages below 220 mg/dL. But between the ages of 45 and 55, women's average cholesterol levels soar to between 240 and 260 mg/dL. Women between 45 and 74 years of age who have a cholesterol level over 240 mg/dL are more than twice as likely to develop coronary heart disease as women with levels below 200 mg/dL.

Total blood cholesterol is the first measurement used to identify persons with high blood cholesterol. As you read above, a blood cholesterol level of 240 or more means you have "high" blood cholesterol. But even "borderline-high" levels (200-239) boost your risk of coronary heart disease. If your total blood cholesterol is in the high or borderline-high category and you have other risk factors for coronary heart disease, your doctor will want a more complete "cholesterol profile" before making a decision about treatment. Specifically, your doctor will measure your LDL and HDL levels after an overnight fast.

Cholesterol travels in the blood in packages called lipoproteins. Cholesterol packaged in low density lipoprotein (LDL) is often called "bad cholesterol" because LDL carries most of the cholesterol in the blood and if not removed, cholesterol and fat can build up in the arteries. Another type of cholesterol, which is packaged in high density lipoprotein (HDL), is known as "good cholesterol." That is because HDL helps remove cholesterol from the blood, preventing it from piling up in the arteries.

A "cholesterol profile" includes measurements of both HDL and LDL levels. An LDL level below 130 mg/dL is desirable. LDL levels of 130-159 mg/dL are "borderline-high." Levels of 160 mg/dL or above mean you have a high risk of developing coronary heart disease. As with total cholesterol, the higher the LDL number, the higher the risk. On the other hand, the lower your HDL number is, the greater your risk for coronary heart disease. Any HDL level below 35 mg/dL is considered too low. After studying your LDL- and HDL-cholesterol levels and other risk factors for coronary heart disease, your doctor may recommend a specific treatment program for you.

For many people, a change in eating habits is the only step needed to lower blood cholesterol levels. Cutting back on foods rich in fat, especially saturated fat, and in cholesterol, can lower both total and LDL-cholesterol. Weight loss for overweight persons also will lower blood cholesterol levels. Losing extra weight, as well as quitting smoking and becoming more active, also may help boost

what's your number?

Blood Cholesterol Levels and Heart Disease Risk

	DESIRABLE	BORDERLINE-HIGH	HIGH
Total Cholesterol	Less than 200	200-239	240 and above
LDL Cholesterol	Less than 130	130-159	160 and above

your HDL-cholesterol levels. Although we don't know for sure that raising HDL levels in this way will reduce the risk of coronary heart disease, these measures are likely to be good for your heart in any case.

While changing the way you eat is the first and most important action you can take to improve your blood cholesterol levels, your doctor may also suggest that you take cholesterol-lowering medications. This recommendation will depend on how much your new diet lowers your blood cholesterol and whether you have any other risk factors for coronary heart disease. If your doctor does prescribe medicines, you must also continue your cholesterol-lowering diet because the combination may allow you to take less medicine. Also, because diet is still the safest treatment, you should always try to lower your cholesterol levels with diet changes before adding medication.

Triglycerides are another type of fat found in the blood and in food. Triglycerides in food are made up of saturated, polyunsaturated, and monounsaturated fats. The liver also produces triglycerides. When alcohol is consumed or when excess calories are taken in, the liver produces more triglycerides.

A number of studies have found that some people with coronary heart disease have high triglyceride levels. However, more research is needed to determine whether high triglycerides cause narrowing of the arteries or are just associated with other risk factors like low levels of HDL-cholesterol and being overweight.

Extremely high levels of triglycerides can cause a dangerous inflammation of the pancreas called pancreatitis.

To reduce blood triglyceride levels, doctors recommend a low-fat, low-calorie diet, weight control, increased exercise, and no alcohol. Occasionally drugs are needed.

*Use this chart to record your progress toward your **healthy heart** goals.*

- **SMOKING**

  QUIT DATE _____

- **CHOLESTEROL**

  DESIRABLE LEVEL: UNDER 200 mg/dL

DATE	LEVEL
_____	_____
_____	_____
_____	_____
_____	_____
_____	_____
_____	_____
_____	_____
_____	_____
_____	_____

heart health

record

● BLOOD PRESSURE

NORMAL: UNDER 140/90 mmHg

DATE	BLOOD PRESSURE
_____	_____
_____	_____
_____	_____
_____	_____
_____	_____
_____	_____
_____	_____
_____	_____
_____	_____
_____	_____

● WEIGHT

GOAL _____

DATE	WEIGHT
_____	_____
_____	_____
_____	_____
_____	_____
_____	_____
_____	_____
_____	_____
_____	_____
_____	_____
_____	_____

other risk factors

Overweight (obesity) is a proven risk factor for cardiovascular diseases. People who are obese — more than 30 percent overweight — are more likely to develop heart-related problems even if they have no other risk factors. According to an important study of cardiovascular diseases called the Framingham Heart Study, overweight in women is linked with coronary heart disease, stroke, congestive heart failure, and death from heart-related causes.

The Framingham Heart Study found that the more overweight a woman was, the higher her risk for heart disease. This was true for women of all ages, but especially for women under age 50. Among women younger than 50, the heaviest group was two and a half times more likely to develop coronary heart disease than the group with desirable weight. Overweight women under age 50 had more than four times the stroke rate of the group with desirable weight.

Overweight contributes not only to cardiovascular diseases, but to other risk factors as well. For example, overweight women under age 50 are three times as likely to develop high blood pressure as women of desirable weight. Overweight

23

what should you weigh?

*Desirable Weights for Women Ages 25 and Over ***

HEIGHT*	SMALL FRAME	MEDIUM FRAME	LARGE FRAME
4' 10"	92 - 98	96 - 107	104 - 119
4' 11"	94 - 101	98 - 110	106 - 122
5' 0"	96 - 104	101 - 113	109 - 125
5' 1"	99 - 107	104 - 116	112 - 128
5' 2"	102 - 110	107 - 119	115 - 131
5' 3"	105 - 113	110 - 122	118 - 134
5' 4"	108 - 116	113 - 126	121 - 138
5' 5"	111 - 119	116 - 130	125 - 142
5' 6"	114 - 123	120 - 135	129 - 146
5' 7"	118 - 127	124 - 139	133 - 150
5' 8"	122 - 131	128 - 143	137 - 154
5' 9"	126 - 135	132 - 147	141 - 158
5' 10"	130 - 140	136 - 151	145 - 163
5' 11"	134 - 144	140 - 155	149 - 168
6' 0"	138 - 148	144 - 159	153 - 173

* While wearing indoor clothing and 2-inch heels

Source: Metropolitan Life
Insurance Company
Actuarial Tables, 1959.

women also are more apt to have high blood cholesterol levels and diabetes. Fortunately, these conditions often can be controlled with weight loss and regular exercise.

What is a healthy weight for you? Currently, there is no exact answer. Researchers are trying to develop better ways to measure healthy weight. In the meantime, here are some guidelines to follow. Check the "What Should You Weigh?" table to find out if your weight is within the range suggested for women of your height. (Ranges are given because women of the same height may have equal amounts of body fat but different amounts of muscle and bone, which affects weight.) Weights above the suggested ranges are thought to be unhealthy for most people.

Research also suggests that body shape as well as weight affects heart health. "Apple-shaped" individuals with extra fat at the waistline may have a higher risk than "pear-shaped" people with heavy hips and thighs. If your waist is larger than the size of your hips, you may have a higher risk for coronary heart disease.

DIABETES

Diabetes, or high blood sugar, is a serious disorder that raises the risk of coronary heart disease. More than 80 percent of people who have diabetes die of some type of cardiovascular disease, usually heart attack. The risk of death from coronary heart disease is doubled in women with diabetes. Compared with nondiabetic women, diabetic women are also more apt to suffer from high blood pressure and high blood cholesterol. Besides helping to cause coronary heart disease, untreated diabetes can contribute to the development of kidney disease, blindness, problems in pregnancy and childbirth, nerve and blood vessel damage, and difficulties in fighting infection.

Diabetes is often called a "woman's disease" because after age 45, about twice as many women as men develop diabetes. The type of diabetes that develops in adulthood is usually "noninsulin-dependent diabetes mellitus," or NIDDM. This type of diabetes, in which the pancreas makes insulin but the body is unable to use it well, is the most common form of the disease. For unknown reasons, the risks of heart disease and heart-related death are higher for diabetic women than for diabetic men.

While there is no cure for diabetes, there are steps one can take to control it. Eighty-five percent of all NIDDM diabetics are at least 20 percent over-weight. It appears that overweight and growing older promote the development of diabetes in certain people. Losing excess weight and boosting physical activity may help postpone or prevent the disease. For lasting weight loss, get regular, brisk exercise and eat a diet that is limited in calories and fat, especially saturated fat.

STRESS

In recent years, we have read and heard much about the connection between stress and coronary heart disease. In particular, we have heard that "type A" behavior — aggressiveness, a need to compete, a constant concern about time — is linked to the development of heart disease. Some studies have shown such a relationship in men. But recent research on type A behavior in women shows no link between this kind of behavior and coronary heart disease.

Another factor that has often been connected to women's heart disease is employment outside the home. The "price of liberation" for working women, according to many media reports, is a high level of stress leading to soaring rates of coronary heart disease. But research from the Framingham Heart Study shows no difference in rates of coronary heart disease between house-wives and employed women.

But it is too early to rule out stress as a risk factor for women. Certainly, some common ways of coping with stress, such as overeating and heavy drinking, are bad for your heart. On the other hand, stress-relieving activities such as exercise can lower your risk of heart disease. Researchers will need to study larger groups of women over time to find out whether certain behaviors, person-ality types, or stressful situations are linked to the development of coronary heart disease in women.

BIRTH CONTROL PILLS

Studies show that women who use high-dose birth control pills (oral contraceptives) are more likely to have a heart attack or a stroke because blood clots are more likely to form in the blood vessels. These risks are lessened once the birth control pill is stopped. Using birth control pills also may worsen the effects of other risk factors, such as smoking, high blood pressure, diabetes, high blood choles-terol, and overweight.

Much of this information comes from studies of birth control pills containing higher doses of hormones than those commonly used today. Still, the risks of using low-dose birth control pills are not fully known. Therefore, if you are now taking any kind of birth control pill or are considering using one, keep these guidelines in mind:

Smoking and "the pill" don't mix. If you smoke cigarettes, stop smoking or choose a different form of birth control. Cigarette smoking boosts the risks of serious cardiovascular problems from birth control pill use, especially the risk of blood clots. This risk increases with age and with the amount smoked. For women over 35, the risk is particularly high. Women who use oral contraceptives should not smoke.

Pay attention to diabetes. Glucose metabolism, or blood sugar, sometimes changes dramatically in women who take birth control pills. Any woman who is diabetic, or has a close relative who is, should have regular blood sugar tests if she takes birth control pills.

Talk with your doctor. If you have a heart defect, if you have suffered a stroke, or if you have any other kind of cardiovascular disease, oral contraceptives may not be a safe choice. Be sure your doctor knows about your condition before prescribing birth control pills for you.

ALCOHOL

Over the last several years, a number of studies have reported that moderate drinkers — those who have one or two drinks per day — are less likely to develop heart disease than people who don't drink any alcohol. Alcohol may help protect against heart disease by raising levels of "good" HDL cholesterol. On the other hand, it may also raise blood pressure which could lead to stroke.

If you are a nondrinker, this is not a recommendation to start using alcohol. And certainly, if you are pregnant or have another health condition that could make alcohol use harmful, you should not drink. But if you're already a moderate drinker, evidence suggests that you may be at a lower risk for heart attack.

But remember, moderation is the key. Heavy drinking can definitely cause heart-related problems. More than two drinks per day can raise blood pressure, and recent research shows that binge drinking can lead to stroke. It is well-known that people who drink heavily on a regular basis have higher rates of heart disease than either moderate drinkers or nondrinkers.

Keep in mind, too, that alcohol provides no nutrients — only extra calories. Most drinks contain 100-200 calories each. Women who are trying to control their weight may want to cut down on alcohol and substitute calorie-free iced tea, mineral water, or seltzer with a squeeze of lemon or lime.

For women, "moderate drinking" is no more than one drink per day, according to the U.S. Dietary Guidelines for Americans.

Count as one drink:

■ *12 ounces of beer*

■ *5 ounces of wine*

■ *1 1/2 ounces of hard liquor (80 proof)*

Source: Dietary Guidelines for Americans, U.S. Department of Agriculture/U.S. Department of Health and Human Services, 1990.

prevention:
a personal project

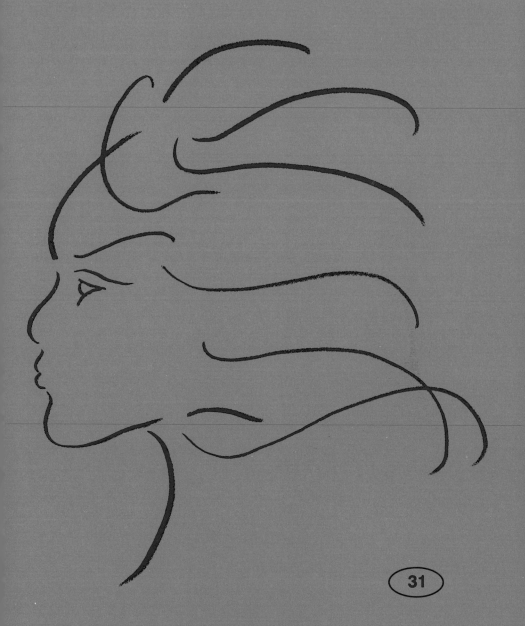

prevention: a personal project

Preventing heart disease, by and large, means making changes in the way we live. For each individual, a healthy heart requires a personal action plan. But where does one begin? A complete medical checkup is a sensible first step.

With the help of your doctor or other health professional, you can find out if you have any cardiovascular disease risk factors, and if so, work out a practical treatment plan. Even if you don't have any risk factors now, you can discuss ways to lessen your chances of developing them. Good communication with your health professional is very important. Choose someone you trust who will listen to your questions, answer them fully, and take your concerns seriously.

But while advice from a health professional is important, the final responsibility for heart health lies with each woman. Only you can make the kinds of lifestyle changes — changes in eating, drinking, smoking, and exercise habits — that will help protect against cardiovascular diseases. To learn about the many organizations and reading materials available to help you, see "Resources for a Healthy Heart." In the meantime, keep reading. The self-help suggestions that follow can help you get started on a personal program for a healthy heart.

to do!

The Healthy Heart Action Plan

■ *Quit smoking*

■ *Cut back on foods high in fat, saturated fat, and cholesterol*

■ *Check blood pressure and blood cholesterol levels*

■ *Get more exercise*

■ *Lose weight if you are overweight*

33

self-help strategies for a healthy heart

KICKING THE SMOKING HABIT

There is nothing easy about giving up cigarettes. But as hard as quitting may be, the results are well worth it. In the first year after stopping smoking, the risk of coronary heart disease drops sharply. It then gradually returns to "normal" —that is, the same risk as someone who never smoked. This means that no matter what your age, quitting will lessen your chances of developing heart disease.

Quitting will also save you money. Over 10 years, a two-pack-a-day smoker can spend more than $7,500 on cigarettes. And that price tag doesn't take into account the extra costs of smoking-related illness, such as doctors' bills, medicines, and lost wages.

Take some time to think about other benefits of being an ex-smoker. Check the reasons that apply to you in the box that follows. Add any others you think are important. This is an important first step in kicking the smoking habit — figuring out for yourself what you have to gain.

why i want
to quit smoking

❑ *I will greatly lessen my chances of having a heart attack or stroke.*

❑ *I will greatly lessen my chances of getting lung cancer, emphysema, and other lung diseases.*

❑ *I will have fewer colds or flu each year.*

❑ *I will have better smelling clothes, hair, breath, home, and car.*

❑ *I will climb stairs and walk without getting out of breath.*

❑ *I will have fewer wrinkles.*

❑ *I will be free of my morning cough.*

❑ *I will reduce the number of coughs, colds, and earaches my children will have.*

❑ *I will have more energy to pursue physical activities I enjoy.*

❑ *I will have more control over my life.*

❑ *I will* _____

❑ *I will* _____

❑ *I will* _____

❑ *I will* _____

Many women fear that if they stop smoking they will gain unwanted weight. But you do not have to gain a lot of weight. Here are the facts:

■ The average weight gain for ex-smokers is only about 5 pounds.

■ Only about 3 percent of women gain a lot of weight (more than 20 pounds) after quitting.

Weight gain may be partly due to changes in the way the body uses calories after smoking stops. Also, some people eat more when quitting because they substitute high-calorie food for cigarettes. Choosing more foods lower in calories and boosting your exercise level will help guard against weight gain. And if you do gain some weight, you can work on losing it after you have become comfortable as a nonsmoker. When you think about the enormous health risks of smoking, the possibility of putting on a few pounds is not a reason to continue.

GETTING READY TO QUIT

Once you decide to stop smoking, a few preparations are in order. Set a target date for quitting — perhaps the first day of a month. Don't choose a time when you know you will be under a lot of stress. To help you stick to your quit date, write the date on the contract that follows and have someone sign it with you. And don't forget to list how you'll reward yourself for becoming an ex-smoker.

Consider asking your contract cosigner — or another friend or family member — to give you special support in your efforts to quit. Plan to get

I WILL QUIT SMOKING ON

_____

     (date)

**I WILL REWARD MYSELF FOR NOT SMOKING
AS FOLLOWS:**

First 3 days of not smoking:

_____

_____

_____

Each week of not smoking:

_____

_____

_____

Each month of not smoking:

_____

_____

_____

Signed by:

_____

Cosigned by:

_____

_____

ex-smoker's

contract

in touch with your supporter regularly to share your progress and to ask for encouragement. Give your "cheerleader" a copy of your list of "Why I Want to Quit" so that he or she can remind you of your goals. If possible, quit with a spouse or a friend.

BREAKING THE HABIT

Surviving "Day One." On the evening before your quit day, "clean house." Throw away all cigarettes, matches, and lighters and give away your ashtrays. Plan some special activities for the next day to keep you busy, such as a long walk, a bike ride, a movie, or an outing with a good friend. Ask family members and friends not to offer you cigarettes or to smoke in front of you. Your goal is to get through that first important day smoke-free. If you succeed on the first day, it will help give you the confidence to succeed on the second — and on each day after that.

Know yourself. To quit successfully, you need to know your personal smoking "triggers." These are the situations and feelings that typically bring on the urge to light up. Some common triggers include drinking coffee, finishing a good meal, watching television, having an alcoholic drink, talking on the phone, or watching someone else smoke. Stress can also be a trigger. Make a list of the situations and feelings that particularly tempt you to smoke. Especially during the first weeks after quitting, try to avoid as many triggers as you can.

Find new habits. Replace "triggers" with new activities that you don't associate with smoking. For example, if you always had a cigarette with a cup of coffee, switch to tea for awhile. If you always smoked at the table after dinner, get up as soon as the meal is over and go out for a walk. If you're feeling tense or angry, try a relaxation exercise such as deep breathing to calm yourself. (Take a slow, deep breath, count to five, and release it. Repeat 10 times.)

Keep busy. Get involved in projects that require you to use your hands: needlework, gardening, jigsaw puzzles. Try out new physical activities that make smoking impossible, such as swimming, jogging, tennis, or aerobic dancing. When you feel the need to put something in your mouth, have low-calorie substitutes on hand, such as vegetable sticks, apple slices, or sugarless gum. Some people find it helpful to inhale on a straw or chew on a toothpick until the urge passes.

Know what to expect. During the first few weeks after quitting, you may experience some temporary withdrawal symptoms, such as headaches, irritability, tiredness, constipation, and trouble concentrating. These symptoms may come and go, and be stronger or weaker on different days. While these feelings are not pleasant, it is important to know that they are signs that your body is recovering from smoking. Most symptoms end within 2 to 4 weeks.

Two things to help you. Nicotine chewing gum and a nicotine patch are both available by prescription. The gum and the patch can help you stay off cigarettes by lessening your withdrawal symptoms. They give you nicotine at a lower, more even dose than your cigarettes did. Gradually, you should chew fewer pieces of the gum each day until you stop using it altogether. Similarly, you gradually use patches with a lower dose of nicotine. Nicotine gum and the nicotine patch are not for everyone — talk to your health professional about using them. Pregnant women, nursing mothers, and people with serious heart problems cannot use them safely. But for those who can, both the gum and the patch can help one "over the hump" and on the road to smoke-free living.

More help is available. There are a number of free or low-cost programs available to help you stop smoking. They include programs offered by local chapters of the American Lung Association and the American Cancer Society (see "Resources for a Healthy Heart"). Other low-cost programs can be found through hospitals, health maintenance organizations (HMOs), workplaces, and community groups. Some programs offer special support groups for women.

Be good to yourself. Get plenty of rest, drink lots of fluids, and eat three balanced, healthful meals per day. If you are not as productive or cheerful as usual during the first several weeks after quitting, don't feel guilty. Give yourself a chance to adjust to your new nonsmoking lifestyle. Ask your friends and family to give you lots of praise for kicking the habit — and don't forget to pat yourself on the back. You are making a major change in your life, and you deserve a lot of credit.

IF YOU "SLIP"

A "slip" means that you have had a small setback and smoked a cigarette after your quit date. Don't worry. It doesn't mean that you've become a smoker again. Most smokers "slip" three to five times before they quit for good. But to get right back on the nonsmoker track, here are some tips:

Don't get discouraged. Having a cigarette or two doesn't mean you have failed. It doesn't mean you can't quit smoking. A slip happens to many, many people who successfully quit. Keep thinking of yourself as a nonsmoker. You are one.

Learn from experience. What was the trigger that made you light up? Were you driving home from work, having a glass of wine at a party, feeling angry at your boss? Think back on the day's events until you remember what the specific trigger was.

Take charge. Make a list of things you will do the next time you are in that particular situation — and other tempting situations as well. Sign a new contract with your support person to show yourself how determined you are to kick the habit. Reread your list of all the reasons you want to quit. You're on your way.

GETTING PHYSICAL

Regular exercise can help you reduce your risk of coronary heart disease. Exercise helps women take off extra pounds, helps to control blood pressure, lessens a diabetic's need for insulin, and boosts the level of "good" HDL-cholesterol.

Some studies also show that being inactive boosts the risk of heart attack.

	WARM UP	TARGET ZONE EXERCISING	COOL DOWN	TOTAL TIME

WEEK 1

Session A	Walk slowly	Then walk briskly	Then walk slowly	
	5 min.	5 min.	5 min.	15 min.
Session B	Repeat above pattern			
Session C	Repeat above pattern			

Continue with at least three exercise sessions during each week of the program.

WEEK 2	Walk slowly 5 min.	Walk briskly 7 min.	Walk slowly 5 min.	17 min.
WEEK 3	Walk slowly 5 min.	Walk briskly 9 min.	Walk slowly 5 min.	19 min.
WEEK 4	Walk slowly 5 min.	Walk briskly 11 min.	Walk slowly 5 min.	21 min.
WEEK 5	Walk slowly 5 min.	Walk briskly 13 min.	Walk slowly 5 min.	23 min.
WEEK 6	Walk slowly 5 min.	Walk briskly 15 min.	Walk slowly 5 min.	25 min.
WEEK 7	Walk slowly 5 min.	Walk briskly 18 min.	Walk slowly 5 min.	28 min.
WEEK 8	Walk slowly 5 min.	Walk briskly 20 min.	Walk slowly 5 min.	30 min.
WEEK 9	Walk slowly 5 min.	Walk briskly 23 min.	Walk slowly 5 min.	33 min.
WEEK 10	Walk slowly 5 min.	Walk briskly 26 min.	Walk slowly 5 min.	36 min.
WEEK 11	Walk slowly 5 min.	Walk briskly 28 min.	Walk slowly 5 min.	38 min.
WEEK 12 AND BEYOND	Walk slowly 5 min.	Walk briskly 30 min.	Walk slowly 5 min.	40 min.

Exercise has many other benefits. It strengthens the lungs, tones the muscles, keeps the joints in good condition, and helps many people cope better with stress.

While many physical activities are fun, only regular, brisk exercise will improve heart health. This is called "aerobic" exercise and includes jogging, swimming, jumping rope, and cross-country skiing. Walking, biking, and dancing can also strengthen your heart, if you do them fast enough and long enough. Choose an activity that you think you will enjoy and that will fit most easily into your schedule.

Most people do not need to see a doctor before they start a gradual, sensible exercise program. Some people, however, should get medical advice. For example, if you have heart trouble or have had a heart attack, if you are over 50 years old and are not used to energetic activity, or if you have a family history of developing heart disease at a young age, check with your doctor before you start.

Once you get started, keep these guidelines in mind:

Go slow. Before each exercise session, allow a 5-minute period of stretching and slow exercise to give your body a chance to "warm up." At the end of your workout, take another 5 minutes to "cool down" with a slower, less energetic exercise pace.

Listen to your body. A certain amount of stiffness is normal at first. But if you hurt a joint or pull a muscle or tendon, stop exercising for several days to avoid more serious injury. Most minor muscle and joint problems can be relieved by rest and over-the-counter painkillers.

Pay attention to warning signals. While exercise can strengthen your heart, some types of activity may worsen existing heart problems. Warning signals include sudden dizziness, cold sweat, paleness, fainting, or pain or pressure in your upper body just after exercising. If you notice any of these signs, stop exercising and call your doctor immediately.

Keep at it. Unless you have to stop exercising for a health reason, stay with your exercise program. If you feel like giving up because you think you're not going as fast or as far as you "should," set smaller, short-term goals for yourself as well as grander ones. If you find yourself becoming bored, try exercising with a friend. Or switch to another activity. The health rewards of regular, brisk exercise are well worth the effort.

EATING FOR HEALTH

The health of your heart has a lot to do with the food you eat. Changing your eating habits according to the Dietary Guidelines for Americans lessens your risk of heart disease in three ways:

■ It helps reduce high blood cholesterol levels.

■ It helps control high blood pressure.

■ It helps take off extra pounds.

As a bonus, the kinds of eating habits that are good for your heart may also help prevent certain types of cancer and a number of other health problems.

dietary guidelines for americans

■ *Eat a variety of foods*

■ *Maintain a healthy weight*

■ *Choose a diet low in fat, saturated fat, and cholesterol*

■ *Choose a diet with plenty of vegetables, fruits, and grain products*

■ *Use sugars only in moderation*

■ *Use salt and sodium only in moderation*

■ *If you drink alcoholic beverages, do so in moderation*

Use these seven guidelines together as you choose a healthful and enjoyable diet.

the healthy diet: back to basics

Each day, choose different foods that you enjoy eating from each of these food groups:

FOOD GROUP	DAILY SERVINGS	WHAT COUNTS AS A SERVING
vegetables	3-5 servings	1 cup raw leafy greens 1/2 cup other vegetables

fruits	2-4 servings	1 medium apple,
		  banana, orange
		1/2 cup fruit—
		  fresh, cooked, canned
		3/4 cup juice

breads, cereals, rice, and pasta	6-11 servings	1 slice bread 1/2 bun or bagel 1 ounce dry cereal 1/2 cup cooked cereal, rice, pasta

milk, yogurt, and cheese	2-3 servings	1 cup milk
		  (skim or low-fat)
		8 ounces low-fat yogurt
		1 1/2 ounces low-fat
		  natural cheese
		2 ounces low-fat
		  processed cheese

meat, poultry, fish, dry beans and peas, eggs, and nuts	2-3 servings	This totals 6 ounces
		  of cooked lean
		  meat, poultry without
		  skin, or fish per day
		Count 1/2 cup
		  cooked beans,
		  1 egg, or 2 Tbs.
		  peanut butter
		  as 1 ounce meat
		(Limit the use of egg
		yolks and organ meats
		since they are high in
		cholesterol.)

Source: Dietary Guidelines for Americans, U.S. Department of Agriculture/U.S. Department of Health and Human Services, 1990.

46

LOWERING BLOOD CHOLESTEROL

Reducing your blood cholesterol level can greatly lessen the chances of developing coronary heart disease. One major study showed that each 1 percent reduction in blood cholesterol produced a 2 percent reduction in the number of heart attacks. This means that if you lower your blood cholesterol by 25 percent, you may cut your risk of heart attack in half.

For most people, blood cholesterol can be lowered by eating less saturated fat, less total fat, and less cholesterol. Cutting down on the fat in your diet also protects your heart another way — by helping you cut back on calories and take off extra pounds.

Today, about 37 percent of the calories in the average American diet come from fat — about 13 percent from saturated fat and 24 percent from monounsaturated and polyunsaturated fat. To lessen your chances of getting coronary heart disease, the total fat in your diet should be no more than 30 percent of the total calories you take in each day. Your 30 percent "fat allowance" should be divided up this way:

■ Saturated fat should make up less than 10 percent of total calories.

■ Polyunsaturated fat should be not more than 10 percent of total calories.

■ Monounsaturated fat should make up 10 to 15 percent of total calories.

In addition, you should eat less than 300 mg of cholesterol per day. This eating pattern is recommended for all healthy Americans ages 2 and over*, and especially for those who want to lower their blood cholesterol levels. Use the guide to choosing low-saturated fat, low-cholesterol foods on page 68-69. If you follow this diet for 3 to 6 months and your blood cholesterol does not drop to a normal level, you may need to cut back still more on saturated fat and cholesterol.

FAT·FINDING

Now, let's get practical. Which foods belong to which categories?

Saturated fat is found mainly in foods that come from animals. Whole milk dairy products such as butter, cheese, milk, cream, and ice cream all contain high amounts of saturated fat. The fat in meat and poultry skin is also loaded with saturated fat. A few vegetable fats — coconut oil, cocoa butter, palm kernel oil, and palm oil — are also

figuring out fat

Your personal "fat allowance" depends on how many calories you take in each day. Remember, the total fat in your diet should be no more than 30 percent of your daily calories, and saturated fat should be no more than 10 percent. The chart below shows the upper limit on total fat and saturated fat grams you should eat, depending on how many calories you consume each day. Check food product labels to find out the number of fat grams (total and saturated) in each serving.

TOTAL CALORIES (Per Day)	TOTAL FAT (in grams)	SATURATED FAT (in grams)
1,600	53 or less	18 or less
2,000	67 or less	22 or less
2,400	80 or less	27 or less

*Source: Report of the Expert Panel on Population Strategies for Blood Cholesterol Reduction, NHLBI, 1990.

high in saturated fat. These fats are sometimes found in cookies, crackers, coffee creamers, whipped toppings, and snack foods. Because fats are invisible in many foods, it is very important to read food labels.

Remember: *Saturated fat boosts your blood cholesterol level more than anything else in your diet.* Eating less saturated fat is the best way to lower your blood cholesterol level.

Unsaturated fat actually helps to lower cholesterol levels when you use it in place of saturated fat. One type is polyunsaturated fat, which is found in many cooking and salad oils, such as safflower, corn, soybean, cottonseed, sesame, and sunflower oils, and in margarine. Another type is monounsaturated fat, which is found in olive and canola oils.

Cholesterol is found only in foods that come from animals. Egg yolks and organ meats (liver, for example) are very high in cholesterol. Meat and poultry have similar amounts of cholesterol.

NOW YOU'RE COOKING

Planning and cooking meals aimed at reducing blood cholesterol don't have to be complicated. Here are a few suggestions:

■ Choose fish, poultry, and lean cuts of meat, and remove fat from meats and skin from chicken before eating. Eat up to 6 ounces per day.

■ Broil, bake, roast, or poach foods rather than fry them.

■ Cut down on sausage, bacon, and processed high-fat cold cuts.

■ Limit organ meats such as liver, kidney, or brains.

■ Instead of whole milk or cream, drink skim or low-fat milk. Try low-fat yogurt in place of sour cream. Use low-fat cheeses. Sherbet or low-fat frozen yogurt can be a delicious replacement for ice cream.

■ Instead of butter, use margarine or liquid vegetable oils high in unsaturated fats. All fats and oils should be used sparingly.

■ Eat egg yolks only in moderation. Egg whites contain no fat or cholesterol and can be eaten often.

■ Eat plenty of fruits and vegetables, as well as cereals, breads, rice, and pasta made from whole grains (for example, rye bread, whole wheat spaghetti, bran cereal). These foods are good sources of starch and fiber, and usually contain no cholesterol and little or no saturated fat.

■ Liquid vegetable oils are a good choice for sautéing vegetables, browning potatoes, popping corn, and for making baked goods, pancakes, and waffles. Use small amounts.

■ Many store-bought baked goods, snacks, and other prepared foods have hidden saturated fats because they are made with lard, butter, cream, coconut oil, or palm oil. Get in the habit of reading product labels, and choose products that are lowest in fat and saturated fat. New baked goods have been developed which contain no cholesterol and very little fat. But keep in mind that they may be high in calories.

For more meal ideas, see "Recipes for a Healthy Heart" and "Meal Planning: A Change of Heart" at the back of this handbook.

CONTROLLING BLOOD PRESSURE

More than half of American women will develop high blood pressure at some point in their lives. Women who have the highest risk include those who are black, have a family history of high blood pressure, are overweight, or have "high-normal" blood pressure. To help keep blood pressure under control, take these steps:

■ Lose weight, if you are overweight.

■ If you drink alcohol, have no more than one drink per day — that means no more than 12 ounces of beer, 5 ounces of wine, or 1 1/2 ounces of hard liquor.

■ Exercise regularly. A regular aerobic exercise program — for example, brisk walking, bicycling, jogging, or swimming — helps weight control and is good for your entire cardiovascular system.

■ Use salt in small amounts, if at all, in cooking and at the table. Try seasoning foods instead with pepper, garlic, ginger, minced onion or green pepper, and lemon juice. Keep in mind that sodium, an ingredient in salt, is "hidden" in many foods such as cured meats, cheese, canned vegetables and soups, frozen dinners, prepared snacks, and condiments such as catsup, soy sauce, pickles, and olives. Check product labels for the amount of sodium in each serving, or buy products labeled "no sodium," or "reduced in sodium."

■ While salt substitutes containing potassium chloride may be useful for some individuals, they can be harmful to people with certain medical conditions. Ask your doctor before trying salt substitutes.

■ If your doctor prescribes medication, take it regularly as directed.

LOSING WEIGHT: FOUR WAYS TO WIN

If you are overweight, taking off pounds can lower the chances of developing cardiovascular disease in several ways. First, since being overweight raises the risk of heart disease, losing weight will directly lower your risk. Secondly, weight loss will also help reduce the risk of developing diabetes and help control it. Third and fourth, shedding pounds can lower both high blood pressure and cholesterol. In fact, if your blood pressure or blood cholesterol count is not too high, weight loss along with other changes in your diet may be the only treatment you will need. But even if medication is required, the more healthful your weight, the less medication you may need.

In a society so concerned about thinness, it may be hard to listen to yet more advice about the need to take off pounds. But too often, women are pressured to lose too much weight and for the wrong reasons: to look better in trendy clothes, to attract male attention, to have today's super-slim athletic look. The aim here is not to promote the false and discouraging idea that "thin is beautiful," but to show the link between reasonable weight and good health — especially the health of your heart.

Weight loss is advised only to reach a healthy weight, not to drop to an extreme level.

Taking off pounds — and especially keeping them off — can be quite a challenge. Here are some suggestions for making weight loss an easier, safer, and more successful process:

Eat for health. Choose a wide variety of low-calorie, nutritious foods in moderate amounts from each food group. Make sure that these foods are low in fat, since fat is the richest source of calories. To make every calorie count cut out snack foods that are high in calories but provide few other nutrients. If you have a lot of weight to lose, ask your doctor, a nutritionist, or registered dietitian to help you develop a sensible, well-balanced plan for gradual weight loss. To lose weight you will need to take in fewer calories than you burn. That means that you must either choose food with fewer calories or boost your physical activity — and preferably, do both.

Keep milk on the menu. Don't cut out dairy products in trying to reduce calories and fat. Dairy products are rich in calcium, a nutrient that is particularly important for women. Instead, choose low-fat, lower calorie dairy products. For instance, if you are used to drinking whole milk, gradually cut back to 2 percent milk, move to 1 percent, and then perhaps to skim milk. This way the calories are reduced while the amount of calcium remains the same.

Beyond dieting. To keep the pounds off, change your basic eating habits rather than simply "go on a diet." Keep a food diary of what, how much, when, and why you eat to help you understand your eating patterns and what affects them.

Learn to recognize social and emotional situations that trigger overeating and figure out ways to cope with them. Set short-term goals at first.

Forget the fads. Tempting as their promises are, fad diets are not the answer. Most provide poor nutrition and cause a number of side effects, especially those with less than 800 calories. Although fad diets can give quick and dramatic results, much of the weight loss is due to water loss. The weight returns quickly once you stop dieting.

Steer clear of diet pills. Studies show that most diet medicines have troublesome side effects and don't work for long-term weight loss.

Get a move on. Although physical activity alone won't take off many pounds, exercise can help burn calories, tone muscles, and control appetite. (It will also give you something to do when you feel that familiar urge for a slice of chocolate fudge cake.) Even moderate activity, such as brisk walking, will burn up calories and help control weight.

Ask for support. Tell your family and friends about your weight-loss plans and let them know how they can be most helpful to you. You might also want to join a self-help group devoted to weight control. These groups provide companionship, support, and practical suggestions on changing eating habits and long-term weight loss.

move it
and
lose it

ACTIVITY	CALORIES BURNED PER HOUR*
SITTING QUIETLY	80
STANDING QUIETLY	95
LIGHT ACTIVITY Office work Cleaning house Playing golf	240
MODERATE ACTIVITY Walking briskly (3.5 mph) Gardening Bicycling (5.5 mph) Dancing	370
STRENUOUS ACTIVITY Jogging (9 min. per mile) Swimming	580
VERY STRENUOUS ACTIVITY Running (7 min. per mile) Racquetball Skiing	740

*For a healthy 140-pound woman. If you weigh more than 140 pounds, you will probably burn more calories per hour. If you weigh less, you will probably burn fewer calories per hour.

Source: Dietary Guidelines for Americans, U.S. Department of Agriculture/ U.S. Department of Health and Human Services, 1990.

55

other prevention issues

HORMONES AND MENOPAUSE

Should menopausal women use "hormone replacement therapy"?

There is no simple answer to this question.

Menopause is caused by a decrease in estrogen and other hormones produced by a woman's ovaries. It happens naturally in most women between the ages of 45 and 55, and it also occurs in any woman whose ovaries are removed by an operation. As estrogen levels begin to drop, some women develop uncomfortable symptoms such as "hot flashes" and mood changes. Hormone replacement therapy — a term for prescription hormone pills that are taken daily — can be used to relieve these symptoms. Some women are prescribed pills that contain only estrogen. Others take estrogen combined with a second hormone called progestin.

Estrogen pills have several important benefits. They can help you feel more comfortable as your body adjusts to lower estrogen levels. They also help to prevent osteoporosis, a thinning of the bones that makes them more likely to break in later life. Many studies also have found that estrogen pills help protect women from developing coronary heart disease, but more research is needed before we will know this for sure.

Estrogen therapy also has risks. It may increase the chances of developing gallbladder disease, and it may worsen migraine headaches. It may also increase the risk of breast cancer. But by far, the biggest risk of taking estrogen pills is cancer of the uterus. Women on estrogen therapy after menopause are up to six times more likely to develop uterine cancer than women not on this treatment. It is important to point out that women are much more likely to die of coronary heart disease than from uterine cancer. Still, the cancer risk exists and must be taken seriously and discussed with your doctor.

Because of the risk of uterine cancer, some doctors now prescribe estrogen in combination with the hormone progestin. When progestin is taken along with estrogen, the risk of cancer of the uterus is reduced. While this is good news, we don't yet know how this newer "combo" treatment affects other aspects of women's health. We don't know, for example, whether the progestin-estrogen combination is a safe and effective way to prevent heart disease. We don't know whether the combined hormones are as successful as estrogen alone in protecting women from osteoporosis. Finally, we don't yet know whether this combination will boost the risk of breast cancer. Studies are now under way to find answers to these important questions.

In the meantime, a woman and her doctor must decide whether the benefits of hormone therapy are worth the risks. If you are considering this treatment, you will need to consider your overall health and your personal and family history of heart disease, uterine and breast cancer, and osteoporosis.

If you are now on hormone therapy, check with your doctor to be sure you are taking the lowest possible effective dose. At least every 6 months, you and your doctor should discuss whether you need to continue treatment. Be alert for signs of trouble — abnormal bleeding, breast lumps, shortness of breath, dizziness, severe headaches, pain in your calves or chest — and report them immediately. See your doctor at least once a year for a physical examination.

THE ASPIRIN QUESTION

You may have heard that taking aspirin regularly can help prevent heart attacks. Is this a good idea for you? Maybe.

A recent study of more than 87,000 women found that those who took a low dose of aspirin regularly were less likely to suffer a first heart attack than women who took no aspirin. Older women appeared to benefit most: those over age 50 had a 32 percent lower risk of heart attack, while women overall had a 25 percent lower risk. While earlier research has shown that aspirin can help prevent heart attacks in men, this was the first study to suggest a similar benefit for women.

Other recent research suggests that only a tiny daily dose of aspirin may be needed to protect against heart attacks. One study found that for both women and men, taking only 30 mg of aspirin daily — one-tenth the strength of a regular aspirin — helped prevent heart attacks as effectively as the usual 300 mg dose. The smaller dose also caused less stomach irritation.

While these recent reports are encouraging, more study is needed before we can be sure that aspirin is safe and effective in preventing heart attacks in women. What is known for sure is that you should not take aspirin to prevent a heart attack without first discussing it with your doctor. Aspirin is a powerful drug with many side effects. It can increase your chances of getting ulcers and stroke from a hemorrhage. Only a doctor who knows your complete medical history and current health can judge whether the benefit you may gain from aspirin outweighs the risks.

research: new focus on women

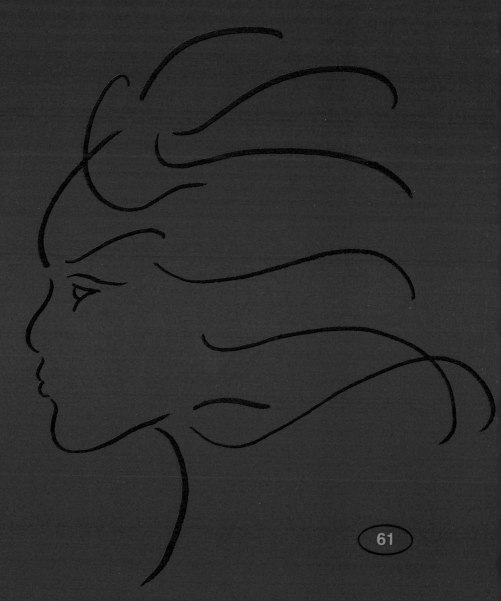

research: new focus on women

As you have read through this handbook, you may have noticed the recurring words: "more research is needed." This is true. Until very recently, men were the main subjects of heart disease research. We now know, however, that coronary heart disease is indeed a woman's concern. We know that we need to understand more about women's heart problems if we are to prevent and treat these problems successfully. As a result, several major research projects are now under way. They include studies on:

- The effects of hormone replacement therapy on cardiovascular diseases, uterine cancer, breast cancer, and osteoporosis. Both estrogen pills and estrogen-progestin combinations are being studied.

- Whether low doses of aspirin can safely and successfully protect women from heart attacks.

- The effect of a low-saturated-fat diet on preventing coronary heart disease in women.

- Whether commonly used programs to encourage exercise, weight control, and quitting smoking are successful for women.

- Possible links between stress, hormonal changes, and risk for coronary heart disease in women.

These and other important research projects will give us new information and tools to better protect

ourselves from coronary heart disease. They will
also help doctors identify and treat women's heart
problems more successfully. Where women's
hearts are concerned, knowledge is power — the
power to improve our health and enrich our lives.

the heart
of the matter

Getting serious about heart health may seem like a huge project. Because it means making basic changes in health and living habits, for many it is a major effort. But it doesn't have to be an overwhelming one. Some people find it easier to tackle only one habit at a time. If you smoke cigarettes and also eat a high-fat diet, for example, work on kicking the smoking habit first. Then, once you have gotten used to life without cigarettes, begin skimming the fat from your diet.

And remember: nobody's perfect. Nobody always eats the ideal diet or gets just the right amount of exercise. Few smokers are able to swear off cigarettes without a slip or two along the way. The important thing is to want to make healthful changes, and then to follow a sensible, realistic plan that will gradually lessen your chances of developing cardiovascular diseases.

Women are taking a more active role in their own health care. We are asking more questions and we are seeking more self-help solutions. We are concerned not only about treatment, but about the prevention of a wide range of health problems. Taking steps to prevent cardiovascular diseases is part of this growing movement to promote and protect personal health. The rewards of a healthy heart are well worth the effort.

meal planning:
a change of heart

AVERAGE AMERICAN DIET (37% FAT)   A NEW LOW-FAT DIET (30% FAT)

BREAKFAST
1 fried egg
2 slices white toast with 1 teaspoon butter
1 cup orange juice

SNACK
1 doughnut

LUNCH
1 grilled cheese (2 ounces)
   sandwich on white bread
2 oatmeal cookies
black coffee or tea

SNACK
20 cheese cracker squares

DINNER
3 ounces fried hamburger with ketchup
1 baked potato with sour cream
3/4 cup steamed broccoli with
   1 teaspoon butter
1 cup whole milk
1 piece frosted marble cake

NUTRIENT ANALYSIS
Calories 2,000
Total fat (percent of calories) 37
Saturated fat (percent of calories) 19
Cholesterol 505 mgs

BREAKFAST
1cup corn flakes with blueberries
1 cup 1% milk
1 slice rye toast with 1 teaspoon margarine
1 cup orange juice
black coffee or tea

SNACK
1 toasted pumpernickel bagel
   with 1 teaspoon margarine

LUNCH
1 tuna salad (3 ounces) sandwich
   on whole wheat bread
   with lettuce and tomato
1 graham cracker
tea with lemon

SNACK
1 crisp apple

DINNER
3 ounces broiled lean ground beef
   with ketchup
1 baked potato with low-fat
   plain yogurt and chives
3/4 cup steamed broccoli with
   1 teaspoon margarine
tossed garden salad with
   1 tablespoon oil and vinegar dressing
1 cup 1% milk
1 small piece homemade gingerbread
   with maraschino cherry and sprig of mint

NUTRIENT ANALYSIS
Calories 2,000
Total fat (percent of calories) 30
Saturated fat (percent of calories) 10
Cholesterol 186 mgs

a guide to choosing low-fat, low-cholesterol foods

Variety is the spice of life. Choose foods every day from each of the following food groups. Choose different foods from within groups, especially foods low in saturated fat and cholesterol (the Choose column). As a guide, the recommended daily number of servings for adults is listed for each food group. But you'll have to decide on the number of servings you need to lose or maintain your weight. If you need help, ask a dietitian or your doctor.

(69)

Source: Adapted from *Report of the Expert Panel on Detection, Evaluation, and Treatment of High Blood Cholesterol in Adults,* NHLBI, 1989.

GO EASY ON	DECREASE
	"Prime" grade *fatty* cuts of meat like: •beef-corned beef brisket, regular ground, short ribs •pork-spareribs, blade roll Goose, domestic duck Organ meats, like: liver, kidney, sweetbreads, brain Sausage • bacon • frankfurters • regular luncheon meats Caviar, roe
2% milk Part-skim ricotta Part-skim or imitation hard cheeses, like: part-skim mozzarella "Light" cream cheese "Light" sour cream	Whole milk, like: regular, evaporated, condensed Cream, half-and-half, most nondairy creamers and products, real or nondairy whipped cream Cream cheese, sour cream, ice cream, custard-style yogurt Whole-milk ricotta High-fat cheese, like: Neufchatel, Brie, Swiss, American, mozzarella, feta, cheddar, Muenster
	Egg yolks
Nuts and seeds Avocados and olives	Butter, coconut oil, palm kernel oil, palm oil, lard, bacon fat Margarine or shortening made with saturated fats listed above Dressings made with egg yolk
Store-bought pancakes, waffles, biscuits, muffins, cornbread	Croissants, butter rolls, sweet rolls, Danish pastry, doughnuts Most snack crackers, like: cheese crackers, butter crackers, those made with saturated fats Granola-type cereals made with saturated fats Pasta and rice prepared with cream, butter, or cheese sauces, egg noodles
	Vegetables prepared in butter, cream, or sauce
Frozen desserts, like: ice milk Homemade cakes, cookies, and pies using unsaturated oils sparingly Fruit crisps and cobblers Potato and corn chips prepared with unsaturated vegetable oil	High-fat frozen desserts, like: ice cream, frozen tofu High-fat cakes, like: most store-bought, pound, and frosted cakes Store-bought pies, most store-bought cookies Most candy, like: chocolate bars Potato and corn chips prepared with saturated fat Buttered popcorn High-fat beverages, like: frappes, milkshakes, floats, eggnogs
	Ingredients Higher in Saturated Fat or Cholesterol: Chocolate Animal fat, like: bacon, beef, ham, lamb, meat, pork, chicken or turkey fats, butter, lard Coconut, coconut oil, palm-kernel or palm oil Cream Egg and egg-yolk solids Hardened fat or oil Hydrogenated vegetable oil Shortening or vegetable shortening, unspecified vegetable oil (could be coconut, palm-kernel, palm)

CHOOSE

**MEAT, POULTRY, FISH
AND SHELLFISH
(up to 6 ounces a day)**

Lean cuts of meat with fat trimmed, like:
- beef-round, sirloin, chuck, loin
- lamb-leg, arm, loin, rib
- pork-tenderloin, leg (fresh), shoulder (arm or picnic)
- veal-all trimmed cuts except ground
- poultry without skin
- fish, shellfish

**DAIRY PRODUCTS
(2 servings a day;
3 servings for women who are
pregnant or breast feeding)**

Skim milk, 1% milk, low-fat buttermilk,
  low-fat evaporated or nonfat milk
Low-fat yogurt and low-fat frozen yogurt
Low-fat soft cheeses, like: cottage, farmer, pot
Cheese labeled no more than 2 to 6 grams of fat an ounce

**EGGS
(no more than 3 egg
yolks a week)**

Egg whites
Cholesterol-free egg substitutes

**FATS AND OILS
(up to 6 to 8
teaspoons a day)**

Unsaturated vegetable oils like: corn, olive, peanut, rapeseed
  (canola oil), safflower, sesame, soybean
Margarine or shortening made with unsaturated fats listed
  above: liquid tub, stick
Diet mayonnaise, salad dressings made with unsaturated
  fats listed above
Low-fat dressings

**BREADS, CEREALS,
PASTA, RICE, DRIED PEAS
AND BEANS
(6 to 11 servings a day)**

Breads, like: white, whole wheat, pumpernickel, and rye breads;
  sandwich buns; dinner rolls; rice cakes
Low-fat crackers, like: matzo, pita; bagels; English muffins;
  bread sticks, rye krisp, saltines, zwieback
Hot cereals, most cold dry cereals
Pasta, like: plain noodles, spaghetti, macaroni
Any grain rice
Dried peas and beans, like: split peas, black-eyed peas,
  chick peas, kidney beans, navy beans, lentils, soybeans,
  soybean curd (tofu)

**FRUITS AND VEGETABLES
(2 to 4 servings of fruit and
3 to 5 servings of vegetables)**

Fresh, frozen, canned, or dried fruits and vegetables

**SWEETS AND SNACKS
(avoid too many sweets)**

Low-fat frozen desserts, like: sherbet, sorbet, Italian ice,
  frozen yogurt, popsicles
Low-fat cakes, like: angel food cake
Low-fat cookies, like: fig bars, gingersnaps
Low-fat candy, like: jelly beans, hard candy
Low-fat snacks, like: plain popcorn, pretzels
Nonfat beverages, like: carbonated drinks, juices, tea, coffee

LABEL INGREDIENTS
To avoid much fat, saturated
fat, or cholesterol, go easy
on products that list first
any fat, oil, or ingredients
higher in saturated fat or
cholesterol. Choose more
often those products that
contain ingredients lower in
saturated fat or cholesterol.

Ingredients Lower in Saturated Fat or Cholesterol:
Carob, cocoa
Oils, like: corn cottonseed, olive, safflower, sesame,
  soybean, sunflower
Nonfat dry milk, nonfat dry milk solids, skim milk

recipes for a healthy heart

1 Tbsp margarine

2 Tbsp finely chopped celery

2 Tbsp finely chopped onion

2 Tbsp finely chopped green pepper

1 10-oz pkg frozen whole kernel corn

1 C peeled, diced, raw potatoes

2 Tbsp chopped fresh parsley

1 C water

1/4 tsp salt

Freshly ground black pepper

1/4 tsp paprika

2 Tbsp flour

2 C low-fat (1%) milk

CORN CHOWDER

Add a mixed green salad, whole grain bread, plus a fruit for a satisfying supper...

Melt margarine in medium saucepan. Add celery, onion, and green pepper and sauté for 2 minutes. Add corn, potatoes, water, salt, pepper, and paprika. Bring to a boil; reduce heat to medium; and cook, covered, about 10 minutes or until potatoes are tender. Place 1/2 cup milk in a jar with tight fitting lid. Add flour and shake vigorously. Add gradually to cooked vegetables and add remaining milk. Cook, stirring constantly, until mixture comes to a boil and thickens. Serve garnished with chopped fresh parsley.

4 servings, 1 cup each

NUTRIENTS PER SERVING

Calories/cup: 182

Total fat: 4 gms

Saturated fat: 1 gm

Polyunsaturated fat: 1 gm

Cholesterol: 5 mgs

Sodium: 236 mgs

HOMEMADE TURKEY SOUP

A good recipe to make ahead and refrigerate or freeze until needed...

6 lb turkey breast

2 medium onions

3 stalks celery

1 tsp dried thyme

1/2 tsp dried rosemary

1/2 tsp dried sage

1 tsp dried basil

1/2 tsp dried marjoram

1/2 tsp dried tarragon

1/2 lb Italian pastina

1/2 tsp salt

Pepper to taste

NUTRIENTS PER SERVING

Calories: 226

Total fat: 5 gms

Saturated fat: 1 gm

Polyunsaturated fat: 1 gm

Cholesterol: 93 mgs

Sodium: 217 mgs

Place turkey breast in a large 6-qt pot. Cover with water (at least 3/4 full). Add peeled onions, cut in large pieces. Wash celery stalks, slice, and add. Simmer covered for about 2 1/2 hours. Remove carcass from pot and cool soup in refrigerator. After cooling, skim off fat. While soup is cooling, remove remaining meat from carcass. Cut into pieces. Add meat to skimmed soup along with herbs and spices. Bring to boil. Add pastina. Continue cooking, low boil, 20 minutes until pastina is done. Serve at once or refrigerate and reheat later.

16 servings, 1 cup each

1 1/2 lb chicken parts (breast, leg, and thigh),
 skinned and fat removed

1/2 C fresh lemon juice

2 Tbsp white wine vinegar

1/2 C fresh sliced lemon peel

3 tsp chopped fresh oregano
 or 1 tsp dried oregano, crushed

1 medium onion, sliced

1/4 tsp salt

Freshly ground black pepper

1/2 tsp paprika

VERY LEMONY CHICKEN

*Serve with wild rice
and barley casserole,
a curly endive salad,
peas, and sorbet...*

Place chicken in a 13x9x2 glass baking dish. Mix lemon juice, vinegar, lemon peel, oregano, and onion. Pour over chicken, cover, and marinate in refrigerator several hours or overnight, turning occasionally. Sprinkle with salt, pepper, and paprika. Cover and bake at 300 degrees for 30 minutes. Uncover and bake 30 minutes more or until done.

4 servings

NUTRIENTS PER SERVING

Calories: 154

Total fat: 5 gms

Saturated fat: 2 gms

Polyunsaturated fat: 1gm

Cholesterol: 63 mgs

Sodium: 202 mgs

BARBECUE CHICKEN

Make this your specialty —
serve with cornbread
and a salad of
distinctive greens...

3 lb chicken parts (breast, leg, and thigh) skinned and fat removed

1 large onion, thinly sliced

3 Tbsp vinegar

3 Tbsp Worcestershire sauce

2 Tbsp brown sugar

Dash of pepper

1 Tbsp hot pepper flakes

1 Tbsp chili powder

1 C chicken stock or broth, fat removed

Place chicken in a 13x9x2 pan. Arrange onion over the top. Mix together vinegar, Worcestershire sauce, brown sugar, pepper, hot pepper flakes, chili powder, and stock. Pour over the chicken and bake at 350 degrees 1 hour or until done. Baste occasionally.

8 servings

NUTRIENTS PER SERVING

Calories: 180

Total fat: 6 gms

Saturated fat: 2 gms

Polyunsaturated fat: 1 gm

Cholesterol: 68 mgs

Sodium: 242 mgs

1 lb white fish (sole, turbot, etc.)

1/4 tsp salt

1/8 tsp freshly ground pepper

1/4 C dry white wine

1/4 C chicken stock or broth, fat removed

1 Tbsp lemon juice

1 Tbsp margarine

2 Tbsp flour

3/4 C low-fat (1%) milk

1/2 C seedless green grapes

FISH VERONIQUE

A classic preparation of delicate white fillets of sole with green grapes in a creamy sauce...

Place fish in a lightly oiled 10x6 flameproof baking dish. Sprinkle with salt and pepper. Mix wine, stock, and lemon juice in small bowl and pour over fish. Cover and bake at 350 degrees for 15 minutes. Melt margarine in small saucepan. Remove from heat and blend in flour. Gradually add milk and cook over moderately low heat, stirring constantly until thickened. Remove fish from oven and pour liquid from baking dish into cream sauce, stirring until blended. Pour sauce over fish and sprinkle with grapes. Broil about 4 inches from heat 5 minutes or until sauce starts to brown.

4 servings

NUTRIENTS PER SERVING

Calories: 148

Total fat: 4 gms

Saturated fat: 1 gm

Polyunsaturated fat: 1 gm

Cholesterol: 53 mgs

Sodium: 316 mgs

STIR-FRIED BEEF AND VEGETABLES

This Japanese-style dish is savory and delicious...

NUTRIENTS PER SERVING

Calories: 187

Total fat: 8 gms

Saturated fat: 2 gms

Polyunsaturated fat: 3 gms

Cholesterol: 35 mgs

Sodium: 215 mgs

2 Tbsp dry red wine

1 Tbsp soy sauce

1/2 tsp sugar

1 1/2 tsp grated, peeled ginger root

1 lb boneless round steak, fat trimmed, and cut across grain into 1 1/2" strips, raw

1 Tbsp corn oil

2 medium onions, each cut into 8 wedges

1/2 lb fresh mushrooms, rinsed, trimmed, and sliced

2 stalks celery, bias cut into 1/4" slices (about 1/2 cup)

2 small green peppers, cut into thin lengthwise strips

1 C water chestnuts, drained and sliced

2 Tbsp cornstarch

1/4 C water

1 Tbsp corn oil

Prepare marinade mixing together wine, soy sauce, sugar, and ginger. Marinate meat in mixture while preparing vegetables. Heat 1 Tbsp oil in large skillet or wok. Stir-fry onions and mushrooms 3 minutes over medium-high heat. Add celery and cook 1 more minute. Add remaining vegetables and cook 2 minutes or until green pepper is tender crisp. Transfer vegetables to warm bowl. Add remaining 1 Tbsp oil to skillet. Stir-fry meat in oil about 2 minutes or until meat loses its pink color. Blend cornstarch and water. Stir into meat. Cook and stir until thickened. Return vegetables to skillet; stir gently and serve.

6 servings

1/2 C plain low-fat (1%) yogurt

1/2 C mayonnaise-type salad dressing

1 Tbsp vinegar

1 tsp salt

1 tsp fresh chopped parsley

2 tsp prepared mustard

1 clove garlic, minced

Freshly ground black pepper

6 C peeled, cooked potatoes, diced (about 4 large)

1 C coarsely chopped celery

1/2 C sliced radishes

1/4 C sliced scallions with tops

PICNIC POTATO SALAD

Excellent new low-fat version of an old favorite and very good with barbecue chicken...

Combine yogurt, salad dressing, vinegar, salt, parsley, mustard, garlic, and pepper in large mixing bowl. Add vegetables; mix well. Refrigerate until serving time. Variation: cauliflower salad — omit radishes and potatoes and substitute 6 cups diced, cooked cauliflower (about 1 lg head).

16 servings, 1/2 cup

NUTRIENTS PER SERVING

Calories: 92

Total fat: 4 gms

Saturated fat: .6 gms

Polyunsaturated fat: 2 gms

Cholesterol: 3 gms

Sodium: 199 mgs

77

ITALIAN VEGETABLE BAKE

Enough colorful vegetables baked together deliciously to feed a crowd...

1 28-oz can whole tomatoes

1/2 lb fresh green beans, sliced

1/2 lb fresh okra, cut into 1/2" pieces or 1/2 10-oz pkg frozen okra

1 medium eggplant, pared and cut into 1" cubes

3/4 C finely chopped green pepper

1 Tbsp chopped fresh oregano leaves, or 1/2 tsp dried oregano, crushed

1 Tbsp chopped fresh basil, or 1 tsp dried basil, crushed

3 7"-long zucchini, cut into 1" cubes

2 Tbsp grated parmesan cheese

1 medium onion, sliced

2 Tbsp lemon juice

NUTRIENTS PER SERVING

Calories: 36

Total fat: .5 gms

Saturated fat: .2 gms

Polyunsaturated fat: .1 gm

Cholesterol: .4 mgs

Sodium: 86 gms

Drain and coarsely chop tomatoes. Reserve liquid. Mix together tomatoes and reserved liquid, onion, green beans, okra, green pepper, lemon juice, and herbs. Cover and bake at 325 degrees for 15 minutes. Mix in zucchini and eggplant and continue baking, covered, 60-70 more minutes or until vegetables are tender. Stir occasionally. Sprinkle top with parmesan cheese just before serving.

18 servings, 1/2 cup

6-oz pkg dried apricots cut into small pieces

2 C water

2 Tbsp margarine

1 C sugar

1 egg, slightly beaten

1 Tbsp freshly grated orange peel

3 1/2 C sifted all-purpose flour

1/2 C nonfat dry milk powder

2 tsp baking powder

1 tsp baking soda

1 tsp salt

1/2 C orange juice

1/2 C chopped pecans

APRICOT-ORANGE BREAD

A moist, rich-tasting bread to round out a light meal...

Preheat over to 350 degrees. Lightly oil two 9x5x3 pans. Cook apricots in water in a covered medium-size saucepan 10 to 15 minutes or until tender but not mushy. Drain; reserve 3/4 cup liquid. Set apricots aside to cool. Cream together margarine and sugar. By hand, beat in egg and orange peel. Sift together flour, dry milk, baking powder, soda, and salt. Add to creamed mixture alternately with reserved apricot liquid and orange juice. Stir apricot pieces and pecans into batter. Turn batter into prepared pans. Bake 40-45 minutes or until bread springs back when lightly touched in center. Cool 5 minutes in pans. Remove from pans and completely cool on wire rack before slicing.

2 loaves, 36 1/2-inch slices

NUTRIENTS PER SERVING

Calories: 97

Total fat: 2 gms

Saturated fat: <1 gm

Polyunsaturated fat: <1 gm

Cholesterol: 6 mgs

Sodium: 113 mgs

RAINBOW FRUIT SALAD

*A new twist to a
back-to-basics favorite...
either a side dish
or dessert...*

1 large mango, peeled and diced

2 C fresh blueberries

2 bananas, sliced

2 C fresh strawberries, halved

2 C seedless grapes

2 nectarines, unpeeled and sliced

1 kiwi fruit, peeled and sliced

HONEY ORANGE SAUCE

1/3 C unsweetened orange juice

2 Tbsp lemon juice

1 1/2 Tbsp honey

1/4 tsp ground ginger

dash of nutmeg

Prepare the fruit. Combine all ingredients
for sauce and mix. Just before serving, pour
Honey Orange Sauce over fruit.

12 servings

NUTRIENTS PER SERVING

Calories: 96

Total fat: 1 gm

Saturated fat : <1 gm

Polyunsaturated fat: <1 gm

Cholesterol: 0 mgs

Sodium: 4 mgs

resources for a healthy heart

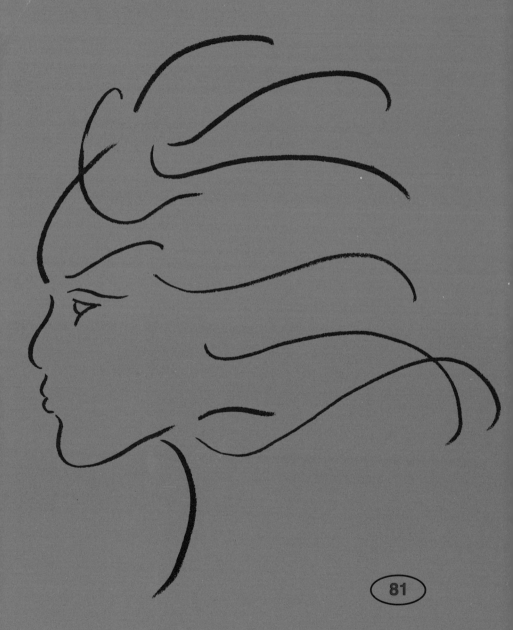

resources for a healthy heart

FEDERAL GOVERNMENT

- *National Heart, Lung, and Blood Institute (NHLBI)*
  Information Center
  NHLBI Information Center
  P.O. Box 30105
  Bethesda, MD 20824-0105
  (301) 951-3260

If you would like more information on the topics discussed in this booklet, the following organizations may be able to help you.

The NHLBI Information Center is a service of the National Heart, Lung, and Blood Institute (NHLBI). It provides public and patient education materials on high blood pressure, cholesterol, smoking, obesity, and heart disease. Publications include: *Facts About High Blood Pressure; Eating to Lower Your High Blood Cholesterol; Check Your Weight and Heart Disease I.Q.; and Check Your Smoking I.Q.: An Important Quiz for Older Smokers.* The NHLBI also offers a number of fact sheets on heart disease-related topics such as *Facts About Coronary Heart Disease.*

A directory of publications is available.

- *Consumer Information Center (CIC)*
  Pueblo, CO 81009

  The Consumer Information Catalog from the CIC lists over 200 free or low-cost booklets on consumer topics. Many are health-related and include booklets on nutrition, foods, exercise, women's health, and smoking. Write for a free copy.

- *Food and Drug Administration (FDA)*
  Office of Consumer Affairs, HFE-88
  5600 Fishers Lane
  Rockville, MD 20857
  (301) 443-3170

  The FDA offers publications on topics such as general drug information, medical devices, and food-related subjects including fiber, fats, sodium, and cholesterol. The FDA also publishes a monthly journal, *FDA Consumer,* which reports on recent developments in the regulation of foods, drugs, and cosmetics. Recent articles have covered topics such as heart bypass surgery, balloon angioplasty, dieting, and nutrition for women. Subscriptions can be ordered through the Consumer Information Catalog listed above. To order materials, contact the FDA at the address above or contact the consumer affairs office nearest you. Copies are available free of charge.

- *Food and Nutrition Information Center (FNIC)*
  National Agricultural Library
  10301 Baltimore Avenue, Room 304
  Beltsville, MD 20705-2351
  (301) 504-5917

The FNIC answers questions concerning food and nutrition and provides database searches, bibliographies, and resource guides on a wide variety of food and nutrition topics.

- *Human Nutrition Information Service (HNIS)*
  Department of Agriculture
  6505 Belcrest Road
  Room 328A
  Hyattsville, MD 20782
  (301) 436-8617

HNIS reports results of research on food consumption, food composition, and dietary guidance in both technical and popular publications. A list of Department of Agriculture publications is available.

- *National Cancer Institute (NCI)*
  Office of Cancer Communications
  Bldg. 31, Room 10A24
  9000 Rockville Pike
  Bethesda, MD 20892
  (800) 4-CANCER; (301) 496-5583

The NCI provides information on how to stop smoking. Publications include: *Why Do You Smoke?* (a self-test); *Clearing the Air: A Guide to Quitting Smoking;* and *Guia Para Dejar de Fumar.* Publications are available free of charge.

- *National Clearinghouse for Alcohol and Drug Abuse Information (NCADI)*
  P.O. Box 2345
  Rockville, MD 20852
  (800) 729-6686; (301) 468-2600

  NCADI is the central point within the Federal Government for current print and audiovisual information about alcohol and other drugs. Publications for women include: *Alcohol Alert #10; Alcohol and Women; Alcohol, Tobacco, and Other Drugs May Harm the Unborn; and Women and Alcohol.* A publications catalog is available.

- *National Diabetes Information Clearinghouse (NDIC)*
  Box NDIC
  9000 Rockville Pike
  Bethesda, MD 20892
  (301) 468-2162

  The NDIC provides information to diabetic patients and provides materials on topics such as diabetes management and treatment, nutrition, dental care, insulin, and self-blood glucose monitoring. Topical bibliographies are produced on subjects such as diet and nutrition, sports and exercise, and pregnancy. A bimonthly newsletter, *Diabetes Dateline,* is also available. Some mailing fees may apply.

- *Office of Disease Prevention and
  Health Promotion
  National Health Information Center (ONHIC)
  P.O. Box 1133
  Washington, DC 20013-1133
  (800) 336-4797; (301) 565-4167*

  The ONHIC helps the public and health profes-
  sionals locate health information through
  identification of health information resources, an
  information and referral system, and publications.
  The ONHIC provides resource guides on a variety
  of health-related topics. A publications list
  is available.

- *Office on Smoking and Health (OSH)
  Center for Chronic Disease Prevention and Health
  Promotion
  Mail Stop K-50
  Centers for Disease Control
  1600 Clifton Road, N.E.
  Atlanta, GA 30333
  (404) 488-5705*

  The Office on Smoking and Health provides infor-
  mation on smoking cessation. Current titles
  include: *Out of the Ashes: Choosing a Method to Quit
  Smoking; At A Glance — The Health Benefits of Smoking
  Cessation: A Report of the Surgeon General; Is Your Baby
  Smoking?;* and a poster, *Pregnant? That's Two Good
  Reasons to Quit.* Single copies are available free
  of charge.

- *Superintendent of Documents*
  U.S. Government Printing Office
  Washington, DC 20402-9352
  (202) 783-3238

The Superintendent of Documents makes available many health-related publications from Government agencies. There are charges for publications. Write for a free copy of *U.S. Government Books and New Books* to receive information on what is available.

VOLUNTARY HEALTH AGENCIES

- *American Cancer Society (ACS)*
  1599 Clifton Road, N.E.
  Atlanta, GA 30329
  (404) 320-3333; (800) ACS-2345

Contact the local chapters or the national office for information. The ACS provides materials, individual and group support, self-help groups, and a speakers bureau. Publications include: *How Can We Reach You?*, which describes risks specific to women who smoke and tips for quitting without weight gain; *Why Start Life Under a Cloud; Eating Smart;* and *Nutrition, Common Sense, and Cancer.* The Taking Control program provides an introduction to a healthful, enjoyable lifestyle that may reduce one's risk of developing cancer. All publications and services are free.

American Diabetes Association
1660 Duke Street
Alexandria, VA 22314
(800) 232-3472; (703) 549-1500

Contact the local chapters or the national office. The group offers patient and family education activities such as educational meetings, weekend retreats, counseling and discussion, self-help, and support groups. Patient education publications include: *Diabetes in the Family; Diabetes: A to Z;* and the *Family Cookbook* series. *Diabetes Forecast,* a monthly magazine, and *Diabetes,* a quarterly newsletter, are available. There are membership fees and costs for some publications.

American Heart Association (AHA)
National Center
7320 Greenville Avenue
Dallas, TX 75231
(214) 373-6300

The AHA provides fact sheets, brochures, and audiovisuals on topics such as general cardiovascular disease risk reduction, exercise, high blood pressure, smoking, and nutrition. Publications include: *What Every Woman Should Know About High Blood Pressure; About Your Heart and Blood Pressure; American Heart Association Diet: An Eating Plan for Healthy Americans; Now You're Cookin': Healthful Recipes to Help Control High Blood Pressure; Eat Well, But Eat Wisely — To Reduce Your Risk of Heart Attack; Exercise and Your Heart;* and more. Write to the national office or the local AHA affiliate nearest to you. Single copies of most publications are free.

- *American Lung Association (ALA)*
  1740 Broadway
  New York, NY 10019
  (212) 315-8700

The ALA and its local affiliates conduct smoking cessation programs and offer a catalog of publications, including many on smoking. *The Stop Smoking, Stay Trim* booklet explains how stopping smoking affects weight and what you can do to prevent weight gain. *Freedom From Smoking in 20 Days* is a self-help quit smoking program. Other publications include: *Q and A of Smoking and Health; Because You Love Your Baby;* and *Facts About Nicotine, Addiction, and Cigarettes.* Contact your local ALA affiliate or write to the above address. Some fees may apply.

PROFESSIONAL ASSOCIATION

- *American Dietetic Association (ADA)*
  216 W. Jackson Blvd., Suite 800
  Chicago, IL 60606
  (312) 899-0040

The ADA offers cookbooks and other materials for consumers designed to educate about food and nutrition. These include: *Lowfat Living: A Guide to Enjoying a Healthful Diet; Food Facts: What You Should Know About Nutrition and Health;* and *Food 3: Eating the Moderate Fat and Cholesterol Way.* Write or call for price information.

The National Center for Nutrition and Dietetics is the public education initiative of the ADA. It sponsors a consumer nutrition hotline that can be reached at (800) 366-1655 (9:00-4:00, central time). Callers can listen to recorded messages on current issues in nutrition or speak to a registered dietitian.